4-4-11

WHERE Doesn't IT HURT?

A Healthcare Solution from a Doctor
and His Equally Frustrated Patient

Thanks for your support.

Merlin Brown

Merlin Brown, MD
Charla L. Sheffield

ISBN: 978-1-59298-381-0
Library of Congress Control Number: 2011920141

Printed in the United States of America
First Printing: 2011
15   14   13   12   11   5   4   3   2   1

Artwork by Shawna Belden.

Beaver's Pond Press, Inc.
7104 Ohms Lane, Suite 101, Edina, MN 55439-2129
(952) 829-8818 • www.BeaversPondPress.com
To order, visit www.BeaversPondBooks.com
or call (800) 901-3480. Reseller discounts available.

I am dedicating this book to my parents: Mom for teaching me how to work hard and Dad for teaching me how to enjoy life. Together you both showed me unconditional love and support. My love and thanks to my three sisters, Marcia, Carol, and Wendy, and my cousin Jan, for their valuable help along the way.

My deepest appreciation to my patients for educating and giving me valuable feedback on the ideas presented in this book.

I wish to thank my partners, Drs. Brunkow, Ivins, Liston, Walcher, and Arthur, as well as my staff for giving me reality checks in developing these ideas.

To Charla, my patient and friend, my thanks for helping me bring this idea to life.

— Merlin Brown, MD

To my husband and best friend, Jeff, I am grateful. To my four beautiful children, Christen and grandbabies, Mama who clapped until her hands hurt, my little sister Shauna for her purity of spirit, and Dad for choosing me to be his daughter. I love you all and thank you for sharing me with my work. I have been blessed to have so much love in my life.

Thank you to all of my family and friends! Chi miigwech!

— Charla Sheffield

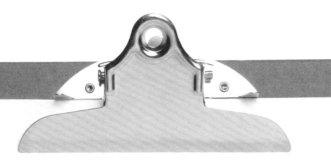

Contents

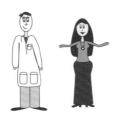

How This Saga Began

In August of 2009, I had an appointment with Dr. Merlin Brown, MD, for a routine pre-op physical. Because I am his patient of fifteen years, our discussion topics quickly covered family updates and landed, as usual, back to the state of healthcare in America. The usual venting on both sides ensued.

At this point, I popped the question, "Why don't you write a book?"

To which he promptly responded with a laugh, "I'm a doctor, not a writer."

To which I replied, "Let's do it together. We have a message that needs to be heard."

Six weeks post-op from my shining new knee replacement, I received a call from Dr. Brown. "You know Charla, I've been thinking about this book. The need is out there. We should do it." My agreement was immediate.

Granted, our patient–doctor collaboration may seem a little unorthodox. In fact, it is. Until we started on the project our relationship was friendly albeit strictly business. A year and many hours of togetherness later, we are friends.

A marketer by trade, I thus had to begin immediate immersion into the inside workings of healthcare. I shadowed his staff, spending endless hours at his office or sharing vegetarian snacks at local restaurants or my kitchen table. We poured over magazine articles and Internet sites seeking both confirming and dissenting opinions on the state of healthcare. We conducted focus groups and gathered patient surveys.

As physician and patient, Merlin and I were *both* veterans and victims of the current healthcare system. We knew we had a legitimate story to tell . . . one that wasn't ours alone, but yours as well.

We certainly had to step outside of our comfort zones to share the information required to make this book important and relevant. However, we truly believe not only in a free market, but also in our country's capacity to fix the inequities that exist.

Dr. Brown's bravery in revealing the inner workings of his private practice and the insurance industry may be applauded by some and criticized by others. To be truthful, at the onset of this creative effort our goal was more to expose the abuse of public trust than to provide a viable solution to what can only be termed a monumental healthcare crisis. Midway through the project, it occurred to us that what the public really needed was not simply titillating inside information regarding the inner workings of healthcare; the public needed a viable solution. We have one, and it did not come from Washington.

My primary role in writing this book was to take Dr. Brown's educated genius and regurgitate it into simple, readable, relatable text. Our ultimate goal is to offer you hope, it does not have to be the pocket-book crippling system it is today.

—Charla Sheffield
(Otherwise Known as the Equally Frustrated Patient)

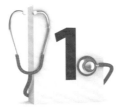

Our Current Healthcare System Exposed

I am going to tell you secrets. Why? Because I have been on the front line of the healthcare crisis for fifteen years and we are losing the war. What you don't know **can**, and will, hurt you. And like you, I want to know **where *doesn't* it hurt?**

My name is Merlin Brown, and I am a medical doctor.

To be specific, I own a thriving practice in an upscale suburb of Minneapolis and specialize in internal medicine. I am a scientist. I care deeply about my patients. By most standards, I am a soft-spoken, conflict-avoiding, logical individual—one not prone to hysterics or over-the-top behavior. Yet, here I am, about to share with you the inside information on a system that, if allowed to go on, could very well bankrupt medical care as you know it.

We cannot pick up a newspaper or listen to the radio without learning that multitudes of American citizens are going broke and losing their homes when catastrophic illness strikes. But did you know doctors are quitting private practice in record numbers? [Source: Harris, Gardiner. "More Doctors Giving Up Private Practice." New York Times, March 25, 2010.]

Think costs are going up and services going down? Take it from a doctor; it is not your imagination. You are spot on. Despite spending more dollars per capita than any other citizen in the world, your choices as a patient and mine as your physician are getting fewer and fewer. To add insult to injury, we as a population die earlier than all other Western industrialized countries! Source: World Health Organization, Source: US Census Bureau, The 2010 Statistical Abstract, International Statistics,

According to the World Health Organization, the United States ranks thirty-seventh worldwide in health. This country was founded on good old-fashioned American ingenuity. You are not happy having worse healthcare than other countries, and I'm not either. We don't want to be just as good, we want to be better.

I know you are interested in this subject, and not just because you picked up this book! I know you are sick with concern because my patients tell me so daily. I, too, am a patient. I have felt the powerless sense of frustration when my employer-based health coverage changed without any input from me. As a business owner who pays for health insurance for a large staff, I have extensive experience in contract negotiations and premium payments—believe me, I delve into the nitty-gritty to find the best policies for the most economical rates.

In the chapters to come, I will provide shocking examples of control and inefficiency heaped on physicians and patients by the private healthcare insurance companies and, better yet, prove that restoring competition would empower you while strengthening the whole system.

You may be thinking, "Dr. Brown, what do you mean? I have many choices. I pick my doctor, hospital, and which insurance plan I want each year." True enough, but what you may not realize is that your doctor's hand is carefully manipulated by the mandates written in the profit-driven boardroom of your own insurance company.

Physicians have much less control than patients realize in determining:

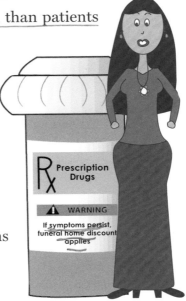

- treatment options
- diagnostic tests
- medications
- hospital stay durations
- preventive health plans
- much, much, much, more!

Surprised to hear these decisions

are not up to the medical professional with twelve-plus years of specialized training?

Let me give you a recent example of our current system at work. "Marilyn," a thirty-six-year-old female, came to my office with lower abdominal pain. After examination, I correctly diagnosed bladder spasms and prescribed **Ditropan**, a drug considered to be safe, reliable, and commonly used to treat this ailment. The insurance company disallowed this prescription, much to the chagrin of my distraught patient. I personally called the insurance company. When asked why we could not get Ditropan approved, the customer service agent simply responded, "My sheet tells me not to approve any drugs that end in 'pan.'"

I am not a politician. I do not believe partisan politics should govern your healthcare options. In my opinion, we have only to examine the national healthcare system of our neighbors to the north to quickly determine that most Americans would be unwilling to sign up for a government-managed healthcare system that could potentially require waiting lists for diagnostic tests or treatment of disease.

Imagine this conversation taking place between doctor and patient: "Mrs. Joy, you have early cancer of the thyroid. The earliest you can begin chemotherapy is ten weeks from now. Fortunately, this is a slow-growing malignancy and you have time."

There are many flaws in our current system. Yet, I have never had to tell a patient to delay treatment due to a waiting list as in the example above, nor would I ever want to! However, it happens over and over again in nations that use national healthcare. That leaves us with the burning question:

> "If the government is not the answer and the current private healthcare system is totally devoid of competition that makes it fair and affordable, what then?"

Life comes with an expiration date, but should we roll over and play dead before our time? Should we keep our mouths closed because insurance companies have all the power? Is half a banana better than no banana at all?

Fear may very well be the most dangerous human emotion. It pushes us into action when it is most dangerous, or worse, it lures us into passivity when action is needed the most.

In 2010, a 2,409-page healthcare legislation bill passed that scared even those of us generally far removed from politics. Most of us still do not understand the words imbedded in those pages. As a doctor, small-business owner, and patient myself, I believe we should be frightened. My ears hear this fear echoed day after day by those I have been entrusted to heal. Admittedly, when Charla Sheffield, a long-term patient of mine, suggested we throw all caution to the wind and put pen to paper, I hesitated in the manner of a man whose life is about discipline and analysis—whistle-blowing is alien to my nature. And, I rationalized, average patients probably don't even understand how out-maneuvered they are by the system; is it my place to enlighten them?

My hesitation was brief because within the reflection came a cure so logical and obvious that it is worth taking personal risks. Our current system is broken and dangerous. Charla and I started this book as an exercise to bring corruption and violation of public trust to the surface. It took a turn very early on and became more about giving hope and presenting a solution to the mess.

Conversations with my patients, staff, and friends led me to understand that in many instances the general public has no idea just how lacking in free enterprise the current system is. In ensuing chapters, I will share the secrets of the trade, so to speak. If you are a healthcare professional, insurance executive, or enlightened politician, the words that follow shouldn't surprise you.

What is a diagnosis without a cure? For years, my patients and I have shared our equally frustrated concerns about the state of our steadily deteriorating system. What we needed was a solution that was not just ideology, but could be implemented to the mutual satisfaction of my patients and both sides of the political fence. In December 2009 (one month after we began this book), while I attended a medical conference in Boston, the beginnings of a true solution hit me:

thats where he was when Christy broke ankle 10-6-09 and she got Bryn woud!

Step #1: We **must** put **competition** back into medicine in order to reduce costs.

Step #2: Eliminating insurance companies from outpatient care altogether would decrease out-of-pocket spending AND allow physicians and patients to decide what preventive measures, drugs, and tests they take.

Healthcare spending accounts (HSAs) already exist, but, in the current form they do not effectively solve our problems. According to the Centers for Medicare and Medicaid Services, 65 percent of healthcare dollars spent are on *outpatient care*. Taking the basic concept of the HSA, I developed a platform that would restore competition, decrease out-of-pocket spending, and put doctors and patients back into the driver's seat of their healthcare planning.

I have coined the phrase, medical savings accounts (MSAs) as the name for the solution that will solve the healthcare crisis.

Could it really be this simple?

I was drawn to internal medicine because I like solving puzzles. Critical thinking is what I do. When my "DUH!" solution came to me, I was shocked at how simple it actually was. It was so simple that I figured something must be missing. So, like any reputable diagnostician, I put it out there to be pondered. I solicited feedback from scores of patients, peers, friends, business executives, and acquaintances, asking for very critical feedback. "Tear it apart," I said. "Where are the hidden flaws to the plan?" Incredibly, approval was unanimous. MSAs would decrease the dollars patients pay out-of-pocket and even allow them to work with their physicians in designing a health plan that would not have to be approved by big brother insurance companies or the government.

An added plus: fees would go down across the board because doctors, labs, and other diagnostic testing would have to compete with one another—imagine that!

Granted, like the prescription bottle in your medicine cabinet, **my plan does come with a warning label or two.** This is not a one-size-fits-all cure to a healthcare system that has been allowed to spin out of control for fifty years. This book will focus primarily on solutions related to outpatient care, where 65 percent of health spending occurs. Let's call it aspirin—not everyone can take it, though most can!

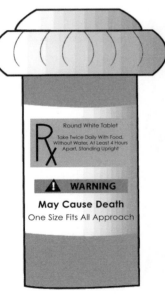

The premise is sound enough to eventually encompass hospitaliztion. No doubt there is a smart politician or two who can recognize the potential and take on the risk

Do you think this kind of change is impossible? Would it involve too many people, changing too many pieces of the puzzle and giving up too many pieces of their own pie? Well, I can't speak for you, but given that our lives could depend on it, I agree with Walt Disney:

"It's kind of fun to do the impossible!"

—Walt Disney

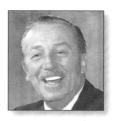

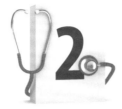

What My Patients Think

As I began to formulate the outline of this book, I received wise counsel from my marketing friend and writing partner, Charla. "Dr. Brown, challenge what you think you know," she cautioned. "Healthcare is a big topic. Find out what patients THINK and what their fears are. Let's do some primary research and get direct feedback from the patients."

I have to admit, as a physician who takes pride in actually *talking* to the eighty diverse men and women in my office each week, I felt pretty certain I knew, in a general sense, what their concerns were. However, always ones to test out a theory or confirm

A Patient's Perspective

> It is critical we challenge our assumptions in regard to patients' understanding of the healthcare system. They are bombarded with conflicting information from insurance companies and employers. It was important that we conducted primary research and got information directly from the source.

a diagnosis, Charla and I created a questionnaire comprising the relevant issue-related topics that came up in conversation day in and day out. We also solicited random patient volunteers to participate in a focus group so we could get their feedback on both the state of healthcare as they know it and my solution or, dare I say, a true "fix."

The survey on the next page is an exact replica of the one given to the focus group. Please, take a moment and test your own knowledge by answering the questions.

A Patient's Perspective

"The patient questionnaire was deliberately simplistic. The issues are complex, but the testing instrument needed to be direct and uncomplicated, straightforward and quantifiable."

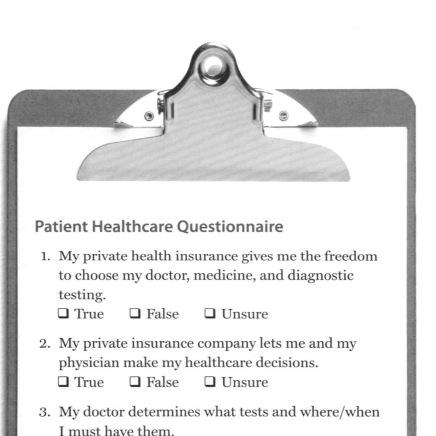

Patient Healthcare Questionnaire

1. My private health insurance gives me the freedom to choose my doctor, medicine, and diagnostic testing.
   ❏ True   ❏ False   ❏ Unsure

2. My private insurance company lets me and my physician make my healthcare decisions.
   ❏ True   ❏ False   ❏ Unsure

3. My doctor determines what tests and where/when I must have them.
   ❏ True   ❏ False   ❏ Unsure

4. My private insurance lets me pick the cheapest options for my family in terms of treatment, supplies, testing, and medications.
   ❏ True   ❏ False   ❏ Unsure

5. Americans spend less on healthcare per person than any other country.
   ❏ True   ❏ False   ❏ Unsure

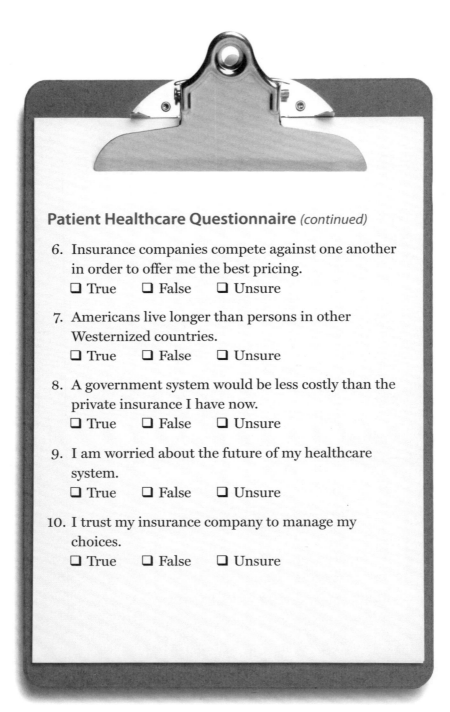

Patient Healthcare Questionnaire *(continued)*

6. Insurance companies compete against one another in order to offer me the best pricing.
   ❑ True   ❑ False   ❑ Unsure

7. Americans live longer than persons in other Westernized countries.
   ❑ True   ❑ False   ❑ Unsure

8. A government system would be less costly than the private insurance I have now.
   ❑ True   ❑ False   ❑ Unsure

9. I am worried about the future of my healthcare system.
   ❑ True   ❑ False   ❑ Unsure

10. I trust my insurance company to manage my choices.
    ❑ True   ❑ False   ❑ Unsure

If you answered FALSE to questions 1–7, you are correct. Questions 8–10 are open to personal opinion, and thus have no clear TRUE or FALSE answers.

Only 38 percent of my patients answered FALSE to all of these questions. Most seemed intuitively to recognize our healthcare is expensive and our life expectancy low compared to other Westernized countries. Yet, a whopping 83 percent did not recognize the extent to which our current private health insurance system is devoid of competition, and that fact alone inherently jeopardizes any doctor's ability to efficiently diagnose, treat, prevent, and cure disease.

There! I have said it out loud! It feels good! No, wait a minute, what am I saying? It feels BAD. Did I go to medical school for an insurance company to tell me what is best for my patients? Are you knowingly signing up to put your life in the hands of business men and women whose professional performance is measured by their profit-and-loss statements?

From the onset of this journey to change healthcare in America, I have stated my solution is bipartisan. I am not playing the blame game here. I am, however, a diagnostician, and the facts support the position that all of us have somehow, incredibly, allowed capitalism to go out the window when it comes to the businesses that encompass the medical industry. The evidence proves that our citizens cannot shop for better pricing or compare a la carte prices.

There is no competition. Unless you have the cash flow of the wealthiest of citizens, choices are limited to the preselected few put in front of you by private insurance plans. Case in point, most medical practices do not have a "real" fee for office visits. Based on agreements with the various insurance companies, a high-side number is billed. It is arbitrary and meaningless.

A typical scenario is this: "Buffy" comes in to her doctor for a routine cold. Her co-pay is $30, which she must pay on the spot. Her insurance company is billed for $100. The insurance company in turn remits $40 to Buffy's doctor, leaving a balance owing of $30. What happens to the remaining balance owed? Nothing.

The golden rule is that insurance companies pay what they want to, no more and no less.

The remaining balance is written off by the practice. To be clear, it is not written off in any *claim-it-on-income-tax* kind of way. It simply goes away, lost in an infinite sea of administrative red tape. As a physician,

Traditionally, American medicine has largely been an industry wherein doctors owned their own small medical clinics. Not so now.

essentially a small business owner, I have no choice but to follow the same rules as my patients: I accept whatever payment the insurance company remits to me.

According to Gardiner Harris of the New York Times, as recently as 2005 two-thirds of medical practices were privately owned. This number has declined to less than 50 percent due to physicians falling prey to the lure of large, monopolistic healthcare organizations who offer salaries that can't be achieved with a private practice. These organizations can afford to pay more because they have more negotiating power with insurance companies. Ultimately, it is the patient who is the big loser: higher cost, less personalized care, and more restriction.

My point is not meant to illustrate the suffering of medical doctors. We make a decent living. My frustration stems from a compromising lack of choice that is as dangerous to patient care as it is unacceptable to free enterprise.

The rest of the test. . . .

My personal responses to the questions are as follows:

Question 8: A government system would be less costly than the private insurance I have now.

Answer: FALSE. Our government is capable of many great things. However, I can cite few examples of when it is more cost efficient than private industry.

Question 9: I am worried about the future of my healthcare system.

Answer: TRUE. If you are not worried about it, you should add it to your list of real things to worry about!

Question 10: My private insurance lets me and my physician make my healthcare decisions.

Answer: FALSE. Don't be lured into fantasyland by the fact that you choose your doctor from a list, which has predetermined your true choice in physicians, drug reimbursements, and medical services.

Are you convinced yet?

The actual case examples that follow are repeated endlessly in medical buildings each day.

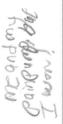

"Jeff," a fifty-year-old diabetic male, came to my office suffering from right ankle pain. The initial x-ray was negative. Anti-inflammatory drugs did not ease his pain. Jeff made repeated visits to my office. I ordered an MRI because I suspected a stress fracture. The insurance company would not issue approval because the original x-ray was "normal." After multiple phone calls and discussions with insurance company screeners, approval was finally granted. The MRI found previously undetected multiple fractures that required surgery.

"Marilyn," a forty-three-year-old female, spent ten days in a rehab center following a full knee replacement. She paid her full deductible of $1,500. Several months later, she received a bill for $353 for an "ice-pack" the insurance company had disallowed during her stay. She was left wondering what kind of ice-pack costs that much money and why was it prescribed if it was not covered by insurance? She was stuck with the bill.

"Ken," an eighty-three-year-old male, came to my office after suffering one year with mucus in his throat, a persistent cough, and postnasal drip. When the initial chest x-ray was normal, his previous physician would not order a CT scan to look deeper. The insurance company rejected my initial order for a CT scan, citing the previous chest x-ray. I argued and received approval. Sadly, my patient was found to have Stage 4 lung cancer and passed away six months later.

You think it can't happen to your family? It happens every day.

Year after year of seeking and receiving patient feedback has left me with a pretty good understanding of their fears and concerns. The results of my patient survey, though well short of a nationwide sampling, I believe are indicative of general perceptions. Some of these are dangerous because they are allowing industry to trample our freedoms.

There are physicians currently experimenting with cash-only practices and even more are walking away from private practice or medicine altogether.

As much as I understand the motivation that drives the behavior, I choose to walk a different path and focus on finding a solution. However, this is one rabbit that will have to be pulled out of the hat by all of us!

"Democracy is finding proximate
solutions to insoluble problems."

—Reinhold Niebuhr

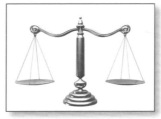

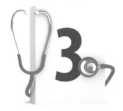

What We Have vs. What We Want

There are two spectrums of healthcare. For the sake of argument, let's say at the far left is universal healthcare. Some term it socialized medicine, state medicine, or public or government-provided medical care. At the far right, we have private healthcare, which includes employer-based private insurance. The majority of Americans have private health insurance. This is generally through an employer who has a "group" policy, through individual purchase, or through the government for programs like Medicare. [Source: Centers for Medicare and Medicaid Services 2009.]

Under the current administration, the term healthcare reform has taken up residence in airwaves across the nation. The definition of what true healthcare reform really means varies in terms of priority, but generally encompasses many health-related issues such as quality, access, cost containment, patient rights, and a plethora of other real and perceived matters.

Because most of us do not remember the days when a doctor traded his service for a chicken, we tend to give at least a passing glance at headlines streaming across the television screen about the dire consequences or betterment to our lives of governmental healthcare bills.

The most curious among us want to fully understand the details buried within the fine print of legislative pages. After all, the bills are written by patriots charged with providing solutions to out-of-control medical costs and inflated insurance company profiteers. The apathetic or beaten-down may feel like they lack any real say anyway, so who cares?

As a medical professional, let me give you some free advice: this is the time to care. This is the time to speak up. Complacency will kill you.

A Patient's Perspective

Charla and I made a few assumptions based upon the fact that you are reading this book. It is likely the business-as-usual healthcare system has hurt you in some way. (After all, where doesn't it hurt?) You no doubt want true healthcare reform that gives you choices and saves you money. You want to be more than a number to your doctor.

> My mother, aunts, and uncles have chronic health conditions. They all expect and dread the day when their doctors no longer take Medicare. My uncle, a retired optometrist, feels like 'strangers' and politicians are deciding how long senior citizens live by limiting their care options. It is frightening how close to reality that scenario already is!

We assume you are an individual who is scared that some-day, if not today, you will need to make a choice between paying a co-pay for a doctor's office visit and paying your water bill. You want to know if there really is such a thing as true healthcare reform. Or, perhaps like millions of senior citizens, you are anxiously dreading the day when the restrictions of Medicare result in less care and even fewer choices.

The other obvious category of reader is big brother: greedy insurance company executives and complacent medical professionals who benefit from a system with more loop-holes than Grandma's afghan. Frankly, this book isn't for them because they already know the half-truths and secrets that are imbedded within the current system.

As a practicing physician, I hear complaints about the current private insur-ance system on a daily basis. My patient base is large and diverse, yet the unhappiness with costs, inefficiency, and lack of choice is common among all demographics.

Q. How can we retrofit the current healthcare system to fit?

A. We cannot.

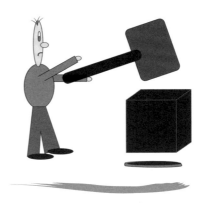

I would be remiss not to men-tion that mixed in with the concern is puzzlement. "Dr. Brown, I don't understand," Mrs. Pruitt states with concern, "it seems like every day I get another letter from my insurance company wanting to 'manage' my prescriptions or help me with my blood pressure. I don't get it. Isn't that what you do? It sure seems like a waste of paper to me."

My patient illustrates the latest trend of bureaucratic oversight currently in the form of accountable care organizations (ACOs), which are designed to limit your personal healthcare and control your doctor. These large administrative bodies take your money (by way of fees charged to your employer) under the auspices of helping you manage your healthcare. To quote President Nixon, "let me make this perfectly clear" regarding ACOs. The ONLY way these third parties will save money is to further fix prices, limit services, and ration care. **Period.**

Unless health maintenance organizations, private insurance companies, and ACOs miraculously invent a way to administer a program without the usual costs of people, paper, and postage, it doesn't take advanced intellect to figure out we, the consumers, are paying for it one way or another. Despite the throngs of letters showing up in my patients' mailboxes and the development of integrating corporate programs, the cost of healthcare continues to rise faster than both inflation and wages.

Third party (private insurance) equals uncontrolled Out-of-Pocket costs. And you can take that to the bank!

The bottom line is this: We are going to pay for any health-care system we have. The meaningful discussion then becomes about what do we want versus what don't we want. When it comes right down to it, most of us want the same things.

What We Do Want

- ☑ Efficiency
- ☑ Minimized cost
- ☑ Freedom to choose: a free market where decisions are made by patient and doctor
- ☑ Quality care

What We Do Not Want

- ⊘ Bureaucratic red tape
- ⊘ High cost
- ⊘ Managed care: healthcare decisions made by third parties
- ⊘ Quality based on profitability

With the assumptions above, does the current private system contain all the attributes it needs to provide Americans with quality individualized medical care? NO.

We have discussed privatization; let's venture on to the left side of the fence to universal health coverage. Forget *For-*

tune 500 companies. **The US government is the largest employer in the country.**

According to www.federaljobs.net, the federal government employs 2 percent of the nation's workforce. Federal employees have some of the best healthcare coverage offered in the private sector, and the average federal worker's pay plus benefits now exceeds $119,982 annually compared to that of the average American worker bee's salary and benefit package of $59,909. With all those highly paid employees, the government must be extremely efficient, wouldn't you say?

Perhaps we should consider the pros and cons of a government-run system.

Pros:

- ☑ Currently, healthcare costs are rising faster than my paycheck. A government-run system would stabilize this.
- ☑ Uninsured and underinsured will have coverage.
- ☑ Preexisting conditions will be covered.
- ☑ A centralized government-owned database is more efficient than private.

Cons:

- ⦸ Does the government do anything efficiently?
- ⦸ A free market encourages competition and reduces costs.

- Government-managed care would further limit choices because costs would be factored in.

- Americans don't like waiting in lines.

- Preventive care options would be restricted; services and treatments would be rationed.

- Medical careers would be less likely to be pursued.

- My personal healthcare info would be in a government database.

A Patient's Perspective

Aren't these negatives of a government run healthcare system remarkably similar to our current private insurance system?

It is not surprising to hear how attracted some of our northern neighbors are to some components of their government-mandated healthcare system. It really would be a luxury to have no out-of-pocket costs associated with going to the doctor or picking up a prescription. You may need to ask yourself if the risks of waiting for a mammogram until you are fifty or waiting months to see a specialist are worth it.

Do not forget the 500-pound gorilla in the room: Healthcare is not free. Under national health-care, it is paid for in the form of higher taxes. With a total absence of competition, there is

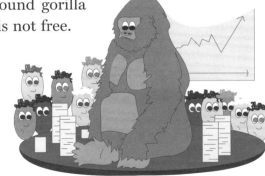

no gatekeeper for cost. This will continue to go up, and your tax rate will rise with it!

Pulling it all together, there are inherent problems with the current private system and the government-managed systems of our European and Canadian peers.

Realities of the Current Private System

- ⊘ Inefficient: wastes money
- ⊘ Fixes price: no free market
- ⊘ Rations care: takes away choices

Realities of a Government-managed System

- ⊘ Inefficient: wastes money
- ⊘ Fixes price: no free market
- ⊘ Rations care: takes away choices

We are on a quest for a meaningful solution. Clearly, by limiting ourselves to either the current private system or government-run healthcare, our worst fears will be realized. Both contain wasteful spending, no real competition, and the pillaging of our freedom of choice by big brother.

"The first rule of any technology used in a business is that automation applied to an efficient operation will magnify the efficiency. The second is that automation applied to an inefficient operation will magnify the inefficiency."

—Bill Gates

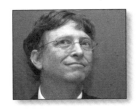

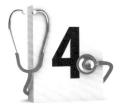

Free Market? I Don't Think So

Americans are robustly proud of our free market. We take pride in our ability to make choices. We compare prices. We look at the ads in the Sunday paper and plan our shopping trips accordingly. If the refrigerator goes out, we may shop at three, four, or more stores before we purchase one that is suitable to our needs in terms of cost, functionality, and other attributes.

Simply put, we demand choices. Manufacturers and retailers know this. Accordingly, they cater to the many needs of consumers who alternately seek economic value, outrageous luxury, or moderation in the products they buy with their hard-earned money. If the market demands it, smart business is there to fill the demand.

Why, then, do we settle for so much less than capitalism when it comes to our own healthcare? Do we not recognize the benefits of a true free market within the system, or is it as simple as an idea that we as a society do not realize that freedom to choose is not an inherent part of the current system?

We would like to think our free market healthcare system is less costly and more efficient than government-run healthcare systems in other countries. Unfortunately, the facts do not hold this hypothesis to be true. On average, we spend twice as much as other westernized countries do on national healthcare programs offering similar quality. We spend $2.5 trillion dollars, or 17 percent of the gross national product, to be well, get well, stay well, and die well. Yet, the costs are still rising more rapidly than the cost of living and income.

Does that mean I am advocating the elimination of private healthcare? Am I saying insured Americans currently do not get quality care? Absolutely not. I am, however, stating unequivocally that our current system, with its complete lack of competition, is not sustainable and will drive us bankrupt.

Q. How many digits in $2.5 trillion dollars?
2,500,000,000,000

A. thirteen

Source: US Centers for Medicare & Medicaid Services, Office of the Actuary. "National Health Statistics Group." www.cms.hhs.gov/NationalHealthExpendData

As a practicing physician, I encounter the lack of free agency at every conceivable juncture. My patients often complain of the same limitations. Based on my experience, I assumed it was common knowledge. When one is forced to make every

A Patient's Perspective

I don't like lists. I want to pick my doctor. Period. I want my doctor to tell me what treatment is best for me. Period. I want to know how much I am spending for services. Period. Why is that unreasonable?

decision based on a list provided by an insurance company, how could it be otherwise?

The alarm bells recently started clanging in my head during the focus group, comprised of a cross-section of patients, conducted for this book. Without exception, the patient participants were smart, interested, capable individuals who were willing to donate a couple hours of their valuable time to share their thoughts and insights with us. The patients represented a cross section of political views, incomes, genders, and ages, accurately mirroring the demo-

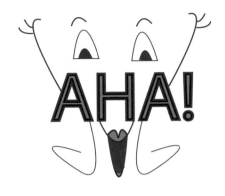

The existing $2.5 trillion system fixes pricing and does not reflect real costs at all. Would it surprise you to hear that in my practice, patients are either overpaying or underpaying for medical services?

graphic makeup of patients in my practice.

The big surprise, the "aha" moment if you will, came after exhaustive discussion and not a single participant identified a lack of competition as a top concern. "Truthfully," voiced sixty-year-old "Darlene," "it just has never occurred to me that I could get a better price or shop around for a doctor that wasn't on my list. I just pay what the insurance company tells me so that I get to have you as my doctor."

Darlene, I am flattered, but in my professional opinion you are getting the raw end of that deal. Our private healthcare system is robbing you of your freedom to choose while stealing the dollars in your pocket.

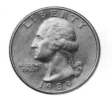

Let me give you a real-life example. Out of my office fee, 60 percent goes to cover overhead: staff health insurance, rent, supplies, payroll, and administrative cost. To break it down further, $147,000 of that overhead is spent annually to process the billing and coding required by insurance companies. On average I get paid $61 for a 15-minute office visit of which I receive 40 percent.

On the other hand, my average insurance reimbursement to visit a patient in the hospital is $63 and has no overhead costs to factor in. It does not take rocket science to figure out that I am either being underpaid for office visits or overpaid at the hospital.

Bear in mind that 65 percent of the dollars you pay to your insurance company for healthcare is allocated to outpatient costs. This may feel counterintuitive to you because it is

Only thirty-five pennies of each dollar are spent on expenses associated with hospitalization.

the huge inpatient hospital bills that so quickly garner the attention of the media. However, relatively few patients are admitted to the hospital each year, either because their treatments can be conducted on an outpatient basis or because they do not meet insurance criteria to be admitted.

As veteran citizens in an active democracy, my guess is that at one time or another you have used ads like the ones you see below to call a plumber, mechanic, or some other much-needed expert to get a quote or bid on a repair. You likely did not settle for the first person who answered the phone or may have even called all three. Why? Because you realized that each business could potentially have different service call fees and by comparing you could find the plumber that was most affordable to you.

Have you ever called your doctor's office and asked how much an office charge would be if you did not have health insurance? If you have, then you realize your doctor's receptionist would stumble and mumble before finally telling you there was no real answer to that. It was a truthful answer.

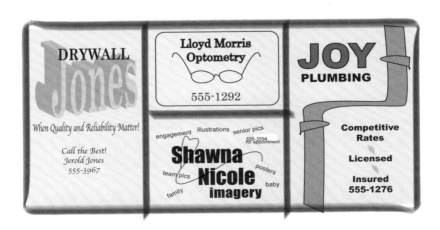

The reality is that a physician's fee for an office visit is not determined by the doctor any more than your co-pays or deductibles are determined by you. Furthermore, the fee varies by person and is not based on actual costs incurred by the physician.

While your plumber and mechanic readily provide service call fees (and incidentally give the same pricing to everyone), no such transparency exists in healthcare. Insurance companies have pre-negotiated rates, and if patients want coverage or doctors want reimbursement, they are forced to sign up. There is no shopping for the best price. There is no good deal to be had.

A Patient's Perspective

This would be like a hardware store telling you what color paint you had to buy, which room you must paint, and how often you could pick up the brush. We would never agree to anything remotely similar to this breech of capitalism at the hardware store. Isn't it baffling that we demand so little when it comes to life and death?

When it comes to pricing, medical service providers simply make the number up!

Yes, you heard me right. It is that arbitrary. The healthcare provider's goal is to bill a high side number that will gain the highest insurance reimbursement. Any balance left over is simply written off and along with it the administrative costs associated with playing the insurance game. You have seen this gamesmanship before.

Each time you open an explanation of benefits (EOB) from your insurance company, you become the chess piece. My guess is you are familiar with the term "allowable" expense?

And further, you have noticed the amount paid inevitably leaves a balance remaining after you have paid your co-payment. This is because both amounts are completely arbitrary and not based on costs. You and I are at the mercy of the insurance companies' financial wizards; in other words, checkmate—you lose.

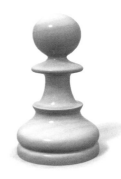

My favorite example of just how screwed up we have allowed the system to become is reflected in our out-of-control costs for diagnostic tests like magnetic resonance imaging (MRIs). In my geographical area, the actual cost of an MRI is roughly $520. Depending on where your insurance company sends you, your plan may pay one, two, or even three times that amount for your MRI. This later data point should not be a *bone of contention* because in a democratic society companies do have the right to determine both their pricing structure and profitability model.

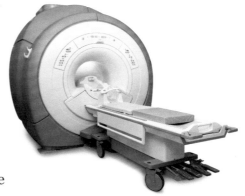

Likewise, consumers/patients should have the right to compare costs from as many medical imaging companies as they would like. A doctor should be able to order a diagnostic test he/she deems medically necessary without "approval" from an insurance company.

That is not taking into consideration that costs are expected to go up at least another 25 percent by 2018. Is your salary going to go up by 25 percent in that amount of time?

[Source: US Centers for Medicare & Medicaid Services, Office of the Actuary. "National Health Statistics Group." www.cms.hhs.gov/NationalHealthExpendData

"To be crystal clear, IF private health insurance did not tell you where you had to go for a diagnostic service like an MRI, a free market would open up and COSTS WOULD GO DOWN for everyone!"

These are just a few examples of how arbitrary existing pricing is for routine office visits and x-rays. Multiply an entire system that functions on this level and you can begin to see why we, as a country, are so inefficiently spending our money. We currently have thirteen digits in our mathematical equation. Annually.

If the past is any indicator, you are not going to get any relief from your employers either. They will continue to pass along rate increases to you. Premiums, co-pays, and deductibles will get larger. The list by which you make your preselected choices will get shorter. Insurance executives will get richer and have no incentive to become more efficient.

Let's look at seventy-four-year-old "Nate." He is a long-standing insomniac with daytime fatigue. After trying many medications, we finally found one that gave him a good night's sleep and improved his daytime fatigue. His new stamina led to increased participation in community activities and exercise. Imagine my horror when the insurance company asked me to take him off the medication because he was "too old."

As any responsible medical practitioner would have, I discussed the situation with Nate. Despite his age, his quality of life was so much better he naturally chose to continue the medication. Counter to what should have been a patient–doctor decision, the insurance company continued, on a monthly basis, to challenge our collective decision to treat this patient in a manner consistent with his best interest.

"Should insurance company policy have the authority to use age as a determinant for coverage?"

At this point, I realize that I am beginning to sound like Dr. Gloom, if not Dr. Death. I don't mean to scare you, even though I, too, feel fear that our system is terminal and gasping for breath. Worse yet, it is letting us down. But we can fix it.

The solution does not begin in the middle by plugging holes or a partisan approach that points fingers.

Sometimes, the cure we need is looking at us right in the face and is so simple we don't recognize it at first. I promise I will get to that, but, as with all illnesses, we have to understand what we have before we can cure it. Stick with me as I continue to unravel the mystery. Have hope. Einstein said it best:

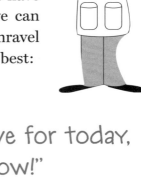

"Learn from yesterday, live for today, hope for tomorrow!"

—Albert Einstein

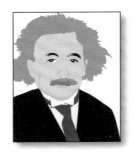

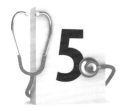

The Cookie-cutter Approach

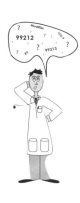

There is a barrier existing between doctor and patient decision making that is both alarming and shameful. It goes far beyond the insult to free enterprise we discussed in Chapter 3. To fully understand the control private insurance companies have over the life-and-death decisions made by your physician on a daily basis, one must first grasp the concepts of medical "coding" and "formularies" and "quality" performance.

CODING. There are five-digit numeric codes attached to every illness, diagnostic test, treatment, and medication. It is called a current procedure terminology (CPT) code. There are specialists in each medical office who carefully (though often manually)

A Patient's Perspective

Prepare yourself. This is a heavy chapter. The good news is if you get this one, you will truly have a deeper understanding of the national predicament we are in. The complications of the coding, quality measurements, and formularies are responsible for driving up costs and pain.

input these codes to a computer system for submission to insurance companies. Once received, they are reviewed and either approved or rejected for payment.

This may sound like a routine and simple business office billing procedure. When taken at face value, CPT coding **does** assist insurance companies with monitoring charts for unnecessary testing and potentially fraudulent billing practices. In a best-case scenario, it can ferret out unscrupulous medical professionals hell-bent on lining their pockets with a few extra dollars. It helps with controlling the use of expired or fraudulent insurance cards by patients, but it does not eliminate it.

However, as they say, the devil is in the details! There is nothing remotely simple about the coding process, and once again we are stuck with a system that is inherently weak, expensive, and arbitrary. Each medical coding book is nearly one thousand pages long and is specific by specialty or discipline; these books are updated each year to reflect new or discontinued conditions and treatments. Each of these codes is assigned an arbitrary reimbursement amount by the insurance companies and can change with each renewal cycle. Human error can and does occur, primarily due to lack of discernment (plans continuously change after all), mistakes, or keystroke errors. The end result is rejected claims, under- or overpayment, and repeated submissions by an already overtaxed process.

Why should you care? Because these system inefficiencies will come back to you either through your wallet or your time. Have you ever received a medical bill that contained an error? With all due respect, if you answered no to this question, I believe you may want to take a closer look at your explanation of benefits.

Let's follow a typical patient chart through the process:

"Marcia," a fifty-five-year-old female diabetic, reports to my office with abdominal pain. After a physical examination, I determine Marcia requires blood work to confirm diagnosis.

Note: Each test has an assigned code and must also be accompanied by an ICD-9-CM code. In layman's terms doctors refer to the ICD-9-CM as a "justification" code because its sole purpose is to confirm or deny medical professionals' rationale in ordering the test. This is how insurance plans manipulate doctors' decisions in ordering diagnostic tests or treatments. (If the insurance plan does not agree with the justification code, the claim will be denied and the patient will be responsible for the cost.)

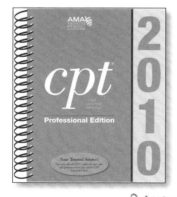

800 pages

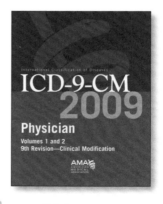

900 pages

Marcia's chart now looks like this:

current procedure terminology

Justification Code

CPT Code	Charge/Test	ICD-9-CM Code
99214	Doctor's Visit	789.09, 250.00, 272.4
85021	Blood Count	789.06 Abdominal Pain
84450	AST	789.06 Abdominal Pain
84075	Alkaline Phos	789.06 Abdominal Pain
82250	Bilirubin	789.06 Abdominal Pain
82947	Glucose	250.00 Diabetes
83036	A1C	250.00Diabetes
80061	Cholesterol	272.4 Hyperlipidemia

Marcia's blood tests come back with abnormal results. I order an ultrasound of her gallbladder. Prior to the procedure, an insurance approval code must be provided.

CPT Code	Charge/Test	ICD-9-CM Code	+ Pre-Approval Code
76700	Ultrasound	789.06	123456

Marcia's abdominal ultrasound is abnormal. I refer her to a specialist for surgery. The coding process starts over again at the next doctor's office.

Unfortunately, in an all too common occurrence...

Marcia's surgeon confirms my diagnosis. However, due to changes in her insurance plan, Marcia's out-of-pocket expense for the surgery is beyond her means. She opts to delay the operation. Two weeks later, she is admitted to the hospital for emergency surgery to remove the diseased organ. She is lucky to be alive.

Once the charges have been processed electronically by the insurance company, one of two things happens. The first occurs when CPT codes and justification codes are approved. The insurance company waits until it has several claims payable to the same medical provider and issues a lump-sum check. Once it is received, an office administrator enters or reviews (by hand) each code and the corresponding payment. For example, #85021 Blood Count $2.23, #84450 AST $1.54, and so on.

Get the picture? This is tedious, painstaking work that is just a keystroke away from mistakes big and small. The average cost to a doctor's office to bill insurance companies is about 7 percent of its revenue. Depending on who you ask, insurance overhead is between 15 and 30 percent. I wonder how many zeros could be eliminated from healthcare costs if we could eliminate coding altogether.

My staff processes bills to more than thirty insurance companies. This means thirty plans paying thirty varying "approved" amounts. Remember in Chapter 2 that I told you fees were literally made up? Line item by line item, this arbitrary cycle

A Patient's Perspective

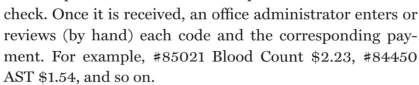

"In my opinion, going to the doctor should be like taking your cat to the vet. You know the charges up front, decide what the treatment should be, and pay as you leave. Why is our care such a mystery?"

is repeated with doctor's fees, lab work, x-rays, and every other service on a regular basis.

I can't tell you how much a fee is because I don't know. The only sure thing is that if you don't have insurance, the bill you will get is larger than anyone else's. Individuals do not get the negotiated insurance pricing. Comforting thought? Probably not, because not only is it unfair, it has no real basis in reality either.

The second alternative is the insurance company rejects the claim. My staff then must recode and resubmit. Very inefficient.

FORMULARIES. A formulary is a list of drugs that your insurance company will pay for. Every insurance plan has one. I do not know how a drug gets on the approved list as there does not seem to be much rhyme or reason to it. Let's look at a couple of real-life examples to see how a formulary could affect you.

"Gerald," a sixty-year-old male with a history of high blood pressure, reports to my office with a sore throat. A throat culture reveals streptococcus, or "strep throat," and he has an abscess. He needs an antibiotic, but is allergic to several. I prescribe Levaquin, a highly effective and, as it turns out, non-formulary expensive drug that will not negatively interact with the medication he takes for his chronic disease.

"Barbara," a sixty-year-old female, has dangerously high blood pressure. She has previously taken several blood pressure drugs from her insurance company's formulary. However, with each one she experienced either an allergic reaction or intolerable side effects. I prescribed Avapro, a proven albeit expensive non-formulary drug. While, in my opinion, it is her best option, at $3 per pill it is cost prohibitive for her.

"Wendy," a seventy-two-year-old female, has long-standing anxiety and has been taking antianxiety medication for thirty years. Her insurance stopped covering the medication so she stopped taking it. Two days later, she ended up in the emergency room with a $2,500 bill for symptoms related to her anxiety. Her antianxiety medication was restarted after I convinced her it was worth it for her to pay for it. Four years later, she has not had another anxiety attack and continues to do well.

"Angela," a fifty-eight-year-old female, is in great shape and has her diabetes in great control. A "health coach" from her insurance company asked me to decrease her diabetic medication as her diabetes was "too well controlled." This is an insurance company's recommendation that clearly even deviates from following standard medical guidelines. Practices of this nature are a violation of public trust!

The patients in the case studies above have illnesses or conditions that require medication. Rejection for non-formulary drugs is an automatic "system" response. You may have experienced this situation. The pharmacist looks apologetic and gives you the "cash" price, which you can't really afford. One of you then calls the doctor's office and asks him/her to initiate an "appeal "and by-the-way Doc, what do I do in the meantime?

Hopefully, your physician can get right on your case and immediately fax a form to your insurance company that outlines the medical necessity for the non-approved drug. It can take the insurance company a few hours or several days to review and issue an exception or confirm the rejection.

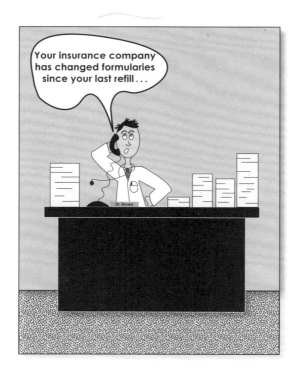

The good doctors take the time to follow the appeal process; the bad doctors look at your formulary and pick a "second best" drug. Isn't that a scary thought?

Meanwhile, Gerald's strep infection and abscess have worsened. He is now in the emergency room because he can't swallow and is in danger of suffocating. Barbara is in the room next to him because she passed out from high blood pressure, hit her head, and has a concussion.

Dramatic? Yes. Fiction? Absolutely not. Day-in and day-out these scenarios are repeated in medical offices across the country.

Failure to allow the doctor and patient to determine the best treatment measure for a medical condition too often results in costly emergency situations that can also be fatal.

Your insurance company regularly changes its formularies. Translated, your ability to continue getting the medication you have been successfully taking for your medical condition is compromised. You know that old expression, "if it's not broke, don't fix it"? Well, once again, unless you can pay out-of-pocket cash, you simply may not have a choice. Looking at the bright side, and admittedly it's a stretch, at least with drugs there is an actual cash price associated, a luxury you cannot find with the remainder of outpatient care.

QUALITY MEASUREMENTS. Merriam-Webster defines "quality" as "a degree of excellence." Using this measure, it is an easy leap to believe if given a choice, most of us would choose to have quality in our personal healthcare choices. In other words, we want our physicians to practice with a high degree of excellence.

On an individual basis, you may measure quality on many levels. Do you feel like your doctor is courteous, listens to your concerns, and takes your symptoms seriously? Are tests ordered that properly identify your illnesses? Are drugs prescribed that cure your sicknesses or reduce future risk for a chronic conditions? Did you feel like you have a partner that is knowledgeable and up to date? These are just a few of the metrics patients use to rate the quality of care they receive.

Doctors are not perfect; they make mistakes and should be held accountable for them. Traditionally, "peer" reviews have been conducted by hospitals and physicians by randomly pulling patient charts and auditing them. This practice continues today and makes the quality checks instituted by the insurance industry redundant.

The Cookie-cutter Approach

Insurance companies also rate physicians and other medical providers using measurement tools, such as reports and audits of patient files. (Please note you have very likely already signed away any rights of privacy that would prohibit the insurance

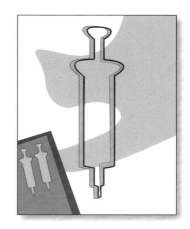

auditors from reading every detail included in your personal file.)

Audits are conducted under the auspices of monitoring the quality of care being provided by your doctor. Every detail of your chart is potentially scrutinized and second-guessed. To put it bluntly, for most physicians, "quality" has become a dirty word synonymous with gouging the patient and doctor for more money.

Unlike an individual assessment based on doctor–patient interaction and strategic planning, insurance providers have turned quality measurements into a cookie-cutter process. They use standard medical practice guidelines (which are not necessarily up-to-date) as the benchmark in determining what medical care they will or will not pay for. Here is a definition of what those guidelines are intended to be used for:

> Practice Guidelines Medical Practice: A set of recommendations for patient management that identifies a specific or range of management strategies.
>
> McGraw-Hill Concise Dictionary of Modern Medicine. © 2002 by McGraw-Hill Companies

Standard medical practice guidelines are intended to be just that: **guidelines**! Their purpose is to form a starting point for diagnosis and treatment. They are not intended to eliminate individualized treatment plans or force substitute diagnostic tools or medications. The definition is deliberately ambiguous to allow the patient and medical professional to jointly determine the optimal course of action.

This is the way it works: Insurance companies will require a doctor's office to pull all files for a patient with a chronic condition such as heart disease or diabetes. The treatment and effectiveness will be graded against a list of the standardized goals/guidelines. These results are tied in to financial reimbursement for the doctor, not the patient. **This is kind of like the salesman of an energy-efficient appliance getting the savings on your energy bill rather than you.**

That may feel a little off-putting because it is you who makes positive lifestyle choices that reduce insurance expenses, but that's the way the cookie crumbles. Let's take a look at a few more real-life examples. Then I will explain how YOU are affected by our current pass/fail system.

"Carol," a fifty-five-year-old female, is a diabetic. In managing her chronic disease, "we" have a list of "insurance goals" to meet: Blood pressure under 130, LDL cholesterol under 100, daily aspirin use, no smoking, yearly urine test, an average blood sugar measurement of A1C less than 8.

Complication: Carol's blood pressure must be maintained at over 130. She gets dizzy and has a history of falling with blood pressures below 130. Although more profitable for me, enforcing standard medical practice guidelines would jeopardize the well-being of my patient. Therefore, because Carol does not meet **all** of the guideline goals as prescribed by the insurance company, I receive a failing grade, which could potentially increase her out-of-pockets costs.

"Allan," a fifty-six-year-old male, is a diabetic with cancer. I met Allan in the hospital. It was his third hospitalization in six months for passing out with low blood sugar. His physician would not adjust his diabetic medication. Allan's oncologist asked me to take over his care due to the frequent falls and hospitalizations from his low blood sugar. I adjusted his medication and his falls ceased. He and his family were ecstatic with his increased quality of life. Allan no longer required the expense of frequent hospitalizations.

Complication: As the physician who deviated from the guidelines, I was given a failing grade and penalized financially for this treatment. At the time of his medication adjustment, the insurance goal for his A1C was under 7. However, the insurance goal has since changed to under 8 due to studies showing mortality was higher in certain patients with an A1C under 7. Could it be that his previous physician had a financial incentive to keep his blood sugar low despite the frequent episodes of hypoglycemia? Or was Allan another victim of the constant moving target which comprises medical guidelines?

"Kelly," a forty-seven-year-old female, has long-standing high blood pressure and now has severe diarrhea. Previously she failed the quality measurements as I have maintained her blood pressure at 140 to avoid dizziness. On her last visit to my office, she had a blood pressure of 70/30, was lightheaded, and could not walk. Her condition was critical, and she was immediately admitted to the hospital.

Complication: I passed the quality measurement easily because her blood pressure was under 130. Isn't that ridiculous? This patient could have died from her low blood pressure!

ISN'T IT BETTER TO "fail" DOING THE RIGHT THING THAN "pass" DOING THE WRONG THING?

"Charles," a seventy-two-year-old smoker with stable coronary artery disease, reported for his annual physical. His weight, cholesterol, blood pressure, and medications were within guidelines. Charles was provided with information on the risks associated with smoking and counseled to quit.

Complication: Charles was provided with information on health risks associated with smoking and advised to quit. Because he did not follow my recommendations, I failed ALL quality measurements.

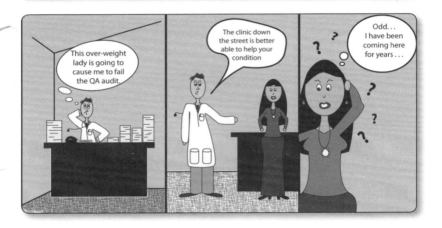

How do quality measurements directly affect you?

When a doctor is put in a higher network "tier" because of failure to meet "quality measures," you will likely have a higher out-of-pocket co-pay. Or perhaps your trusted

As shocking as it sounds, if your condition warrants treatment outside the guidelines, your doctor has a financial incentive to provide inappropriate care.

healthcare partner will disappear from your approved provider list altogether, either by choice or not.

"Jim," a fifty-three-year-old male with diabetes has severe liver disease and high cholesterol. He cannot take cholesterol-lowering drugs because they may worsen his liver disease.

Complication: The quality system currently in place would offer me a financial incentive to prescribe Jim with a cholesterol-lowering drug despite potentially fatal consequences. Insanity.

"Christopher" a sixty-year-old gentleman who had developed a growth on his cheek. He was repeatedly treated by his primary care physician with liquid nitrogen for over a year, but the growth continued to come back. He repeatedly asked for a referral to a dermatologist but was never given one.

Complication: After my first examination with this patient, I suspected skin cancer and referred him to a dermatologist. He went on to require multiple surgeries, including plastic surgery for reconstruction to remove skin cancer and make his cheek look normal again. Could it be that his primary care physician would not refer him because he was financially incented NOT TO?

As I stated previously, doctors are getting frustrated and walking away from private practice in large numbers. As if stifling qualified expertise and killing innovation were not enough, the measuring and reporting of quality goals are expensive and time consuming for the entire staff, pushing medical costs for everyone exponentially higher every year.

Have you ever been referred to another doctor or specialist due to your condition being too complicated? There are often legitimate reasons for referrals of this nature. Perhaps a patient's illness could better be addressed by a specialist. However, in some cases morbidly obese or otherwise very at-risk patients are being sent on their way because of the unwillingness of a physician to take the quality measurement hit the condition would bring. I have never done this, nor would I ever do it. Unfortunately, the reality is there is a price associated with high-risk patients that some doctors are just unwilling to pay.

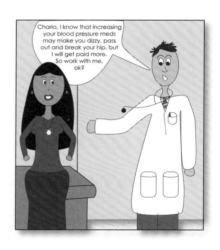

The flip side of the coin is potentially even worse than hurting our collective pocketbooks or our feelings.

Just venting…

Have you ever called a doctor's office and been told there were no appointments available until next week or month? If you answer no, you number among the lucky. The time it takes matching up CPT/ICD-9-CM codes for billing, filling out forms to request an approval for disallowed medication or tests, or arranging reports for quality measurements to be sent to the insurance company takes away from patient time.

There will always be physicians around who willingly comply with standardized second-rate treatment plans and formularies. Believe me when I say there are doctors who are too lazy to fight for you or are lured in by financial incentives provided by insurance companies.

Eliminate coding, billing, and quality measurements and your doctor's schedule just opened up. You may think that is just wishful thinking, but I believe it is a goal within our grasp.

As a physician, I hold myself to the highest standards, and at the very core of my code of medical ethics is primum non nocere: first, do no harm.

My primary fiduciary responsibility is to my patients. The reality that I am required to issue reports and allow their privacy to be invaded by profit-driven insurance companies frankly disgusts me.

When there is evidence to support that spending millions of dollars a year auditing patient files results in improved care, I will welcome the intrusion and expense. I have a medical license, a medical degree, and certification from the American Board of Internal Medicine. If, after all of that, I still require an insurance company to look over my shoulder to ensure your excellence of care, you had better run out of my office!

"In the sick room, ten cents' worth of human understanding equals ten dollars' worth of medical science."

—Martin H. Fischer

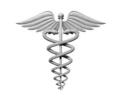

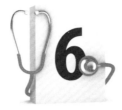

Summarizing the Pain

The short version of what we have talked about so far:

1. Costs for medical care are going up, and services are going down...way down.

2. We have to put competition back into medicine if we want to reduce cost. Our current private health insurance system is devoid of competition and jeopardizes a doctor's ability to efficiently diagnose, treat, prevent, and cure disease.

3. Your healthcare decisions are mandated by in-network/out-network lists and formularies despite what could be in your best interest. Doctor–patient privilege is stripped and determined by profit-driven third parties.

4. Medical coding accounts for significant financial costs for all parties. It is a cumbersome and error-prone system that can result in under- or overpayment and is used to manipulate medical care.

5. In my opinion, national healthcare is not the answer most Americans are looking for. While capable of

many great things, few governmental processes are efficient and guarantee individual choice.

6. You have NO privacy when it comes to your insurance company. Any privacy you did have is signed away when you walk into the physician's office.

7. Your doctor is audited by insurance companies in a pass/fail system and given an arbitrary rating on quality performance. Your chart is scrutinized. Based on the audit outcome, doctors are given "bonuses" or put in higher out-of-pocket network tiers resulting in either higher costs or inappropriate treatment.

8. THE CURRENT SYSTEM IS FAILING US.

The solution to the American healthcare crisis is not retro-fitting the current system, nor is it socialized medicine!

"The right way to reign in healthcare costs is not by applying more government and more controls and making it more like the post office, it's by making it more like a consumer-driven market."

—Mitt Romney

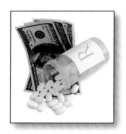

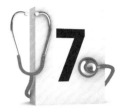

A Cure, Not a Bandage

Y ou have been very patiently waiting for our solution; it is a simple one: Eliminate private insurance for outpatient care, and replace it with a medical savings account system based on a free market.

I hear the collective gasp! Insurance companies and special interest lobbyists are choking on their morning coffee. You may even be thinking I have lost my mind. How can anyone afford not to have insurance?! Yes, this is a radical change to the status quo. However, I am not attempting, as the politicians do, to "retrofit" the current tedious and cumbersome system.... I learned early on in medical school that sugar pills don't cure disease. And no, I am not suggesting we implement national healthcare or send patients with no money out to die.

Let me be clear, if insurance ceased to exist for out-patient care, your life would likely be easier, not to mention potentially longer.

Out-patient Health Insurance

I am simply saying there is a solution to our current crisis we have not explored properly.

Benefits of Starting from Scratch!

The financial and personal benefits of cutting out insurance companies from outpatient care would positively affect not only the patients; physicians; ancillary medical providers such as labs, tests, and medical goods; but also your company's costs. It is not a stretch to state that bringing a free market to medicine will reduce costs all across the industry. Remember the $520 MRI scan that insurance companies are reimbursing up to $1,400 for? In a free market, the reimbursement would likely go down. This is a logical conclusion based upon the fact that technology costs are going down even while quality is going up.

At this moment, put the "how" we could implement such a drastic change out of your head and let's focus on the results of such a plan.

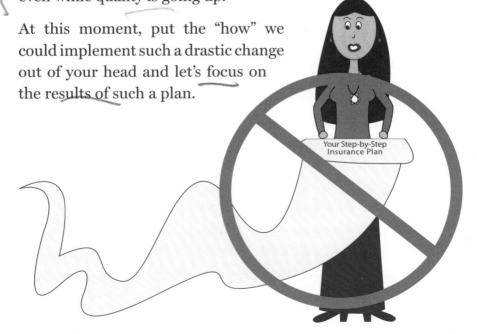

Your Step-by-Step Insurance Plan

Let's take a look at specific examples of the benefits:

- Patients and their doctors would be the only ones involved in decision making for testing, treatment, and medication.

- There would be no restrictive physician lists or drug formularies.

- There would be no restrictions for preventive care, wellness programs, and nontraditional treatment options.

- Physicians will no longer turn away patients due to the type of medical insurance or medical condition they have.(Hurrah for Medicare patients!)

- Goodbye to restrictions for preexisting conditions.

- Medical coding would be gone.

- Billing would be gone.

- Insurance approval to have prescribed tests, procedures, and medication would be gone.

- Insurance approval for referral to a specialist would be gone.

- Hospitalizations will go down because patients would have more freedom to choose preventive and early diagnostic care.

- Competition between medical professionals, testing, and medications would be restored, prices will go down, and quality will go up!

- Insurance-mandated quality measurements will disappear even as your privacy is restored!

- Administrative costs will be reduced for everyone.
- The "bad" doctors would not have enough business to stay in business!

We are not talking about fixing the system with a bandage. Major surgery will be required.

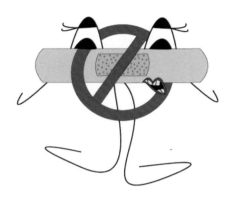

In the chapters to come we will take a closer look at the solution, benefits, and the risks of executing a plan that will bar big business from interfering with your healthcare.

"If all we're doing is adding more people to a broken system then costs will continue to skyrocket, and eventually somebody is going to be bankrupt, whether it's the federal government, state governments, businesses, or individual families."

—President Barack Obama

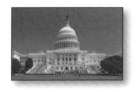

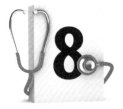

MSA Dr. Brown's Way

The costs of your healthcare will never miraculously just go away despite any political propaganda you may have heard recently. My plan will not be "free" either. I can assure you, though, for everyone it will be at least as good as their current private employer-based system. **For most people, it will be better.** It can also be adjusted to fit Medicare and perhaps even government-subsidized programs like Medicaid.

Step One: Eliminate private outpatient health insurance.

Step Two: Replace private insurance with a healthcare spending account debit card system.

Here is how it would work:

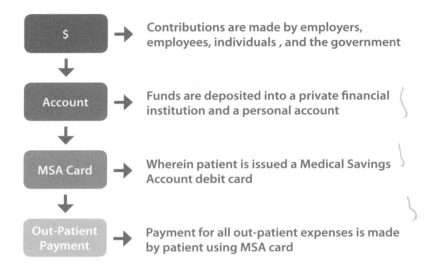

This concept is very different for us. We need to look closely at each aspect of the system.

$ Private health insurance is currently paid for through a combination of employer and employee contributions. Generally, the employer selects a health-care plan (or plans) that provide the most value for the lowest cost to the company. To be fair, I am sure many companies are diligent in their efforts to find plans that minimize out-of-pocket costs. However, all contract negotiations are managed by employers, and subsequently, your choices and costs are as well. Don't forget, profit-driven insurance companies also limit employers' options.

Under the new plan, employers and employees will continue to pay insurance premiums. However, roughly 35 percent of the premium will go to a private inpatient insurance plan (for major medical/in-patient) and the remaining 65 percent will go into your personalized medical savings account.

This model is also applicable to Medicare participants. Currently, the Social Security Administration pays for the major medical/in-patient portion of the coverage premium. It would continue to do so.

In utilizing the medical spending account, employers will recognize an immediate increase in profits due to the elimination of administrative fees associated with billing, coding, insurance fraud, and processing. This same benefit would naturally apply to insurance companies though it is unlikely to offset the profits they will be losing from bloated insurance premiums.

Account The funds paid by the employer/employee/Social Security Administration contribution as described above will be deposited into an MSA at the private financial institution of choice. Similar to a social security number, each person in the United States will be given an account number that stays with them for life. Until the age of eighteen, children will receive coverage under their parent's MSA number.

The funds will accumulate interest, and unlike some current HSAs, any balance remaining at the end of a calendar year will carry over ad infinitum. The funds contributed will be retained for an individual's sole use. A relatively healthy person could reasonably retire with many thousands of dollars in her account and have a solid financial cushion as she ages.

Financial institutions will be responsible for the administration and transmission of funds in the accounts. They will issue monthly statements and provide electronic payment just as they currently do for debit and credit cards. The money in your account will be FDIC insured.

Please note that a secondary benefit of this free enterprise system would be the boost of dollars gathering interest in the financial institutions. Upon the account holder's death, any money remaining in an account will be deposited back into the system for use to subsidize overspent accounts or the uninsured—but, more on this aspect later.

MSA Card MSA numbers will be issued to persons over eighteen years of age. We have considered various scenarios for whom the issuing party should be and have concluded this role is best suited for the federal government. Again, similar to a social security number that remains intact for life, the MSA number issuance should be regulated to avoid fraud and ensure system integrity.

However, it will be the responsibility of the chosen financial institution to issue the actual debit card. It would have an electronic strip for processing and all the fraud prevention attributes other credit/debit cards have. The patient will have the freedom to change from one financial institution to another. Similar to existing HSAs, guidelines will have to be established to maintain and monitor compliance. First and foremost, the funds in this account must be used for outpatient medical care only.

Out-patient Payment

Upon leaving a medical appointment, you will pay for the services received using your MSA card. Unlike the current system, you will be provided with an itemized statement of fees and charges at checkout. Using personalized, market-driven profit models, physicians, diagnostic centers, labs, and other medical entities will be forced to engage in a free market. The process is completely transparent.

Every bona fide medical professional will be able to process the MSA card. You may seek healthcare from any medical professional; there will be no formularies, networks, or approvals required.

COULD THIS Really WORK?

You bet it could. Would it be easy? No way. Would it be worth the pain? Absolutely.

You no doubt have a million questions of "how?" and "what if?" at this point. There are many devil-in-the-detail remedies that will require experts and specialists to identify and conquer. However, I can state unequivocally that my solution, or some version of it, would offer stimulation to our economy that is simply a pipe dream today.

This plan sounds simple, but it truly addresses every issue involved in how we spend money for healthcare. I would like the United States to finally have a private system that delivers high quality without excessive and irresponsible costs for our citizens.

Health insurance should function like homeowners' insurance. We buy it simply to cover catastrophic events like fires, floods, and tornados. All other expenses are covered by the homeowner on a cash basis. Would you ask your insurance agent to write you a check for a broken ceiling fan? Likewise, private healthcare insurance should be reserved for the catastrophic illnesses you encounter. The rest of your money should be at the tip of your fingers by way of the MSA debit card.

I am not ashamed to admit that I want only my patients and myself to be in charge of their healthcare decisions. I resent insurance companies forcing me to allow invasion of my patients' privacy, as they [insurance companies] peruse every intimate detail in the charts. I want to reward successes and do away with a pass/fail system that leaves no room for discretion. It is my responsibility to prescribe drugs and therapies that provide the best outcomes for my patients. Mine alone.

Let's look at "Haylea," a fifty-five-year-old diabetic on a fixed income. Due to medical necessity, she is already on two inexpensive diabetic medicines. Despite my best efforts, her blood sugars continue to rise, and I need to add a third, more expensive medication to treat her condition most effectively. Uh-oh. Big problem. Haylea's insurance company will only cover a small portion of the cost for the new drug. She is now forced to choose between buying drugs she can't afford or continue to let her diabetes get worse. It is a fact, not a scare tactic, to state that should she not choose the medication it could cost her literally an arm and a leg.

The question all of us should be asking is why are cheaper, generic drugs systematically covered (and therefore forced on us)? Sometimes other more expensive options are more effective. It tells me the people in charge of the formularies are either more interested in short-term profits or don't bother to keep up on the benefits and research of "new" drugs. It is a public shame in either case.

Preventive care should be embraced rather than restricted. Under my MSA plan there will be no restrictions on how often you can see your physician. Deductibles and co-pays have gone away. If you have high blood pressure, go to the doctor now versus next week when you have a stroke and need hospitalization. This may seem like common sense, but due to co-pays and deductibles, treatable illness results in hospitalization and death thousands of times annually. When patients believe they can't afford to go to the doctor, they put it off.

"Without hard work,
nothing grows but weeds."

—Gordon B. Hinckley

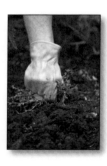

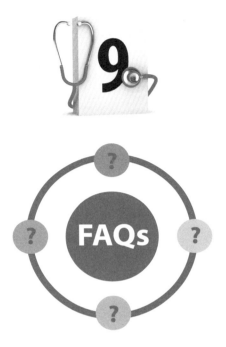

I know you have a lot of questions. How could you not? Charla and I named this book with deliberation. *Where Doesn't It Hurt?* is a title that describes a heretofore helpless and hapless medical system that leaves doctors AND their equally frustrated patients scratching their heads in utter dismay. Today, right this minute, there are many more questions than answers on most facets of the health-care system. If it were easy I would like to think Washington would have come up with a solution that didn't entail thousands of pages of convoluted detail.

While we have done our best to provide a solution that is beautiful in its simplicity, there are many nuances that have yet to be identified or solved. Through focus groups and reader feedback we have compiled a list of the most frequently asked questions.

"What happens if I run out of money in my MSA?"

—Alicia C., St. Petersburg, FL

Truthfully, most people will not run out of money. The use-it-or-lose-it component of many healthcare spending accounts goes away as will overhead and fraud—saving 5 percent to 25 percent of the cost right off the top. A free market will result in lowered prices for the first time in many years; medical professionals will be competing for your dollar. Also, interest-bearing funds within your account will accumulate over time and "healthy" years will supplement times when you dip into the fund. For the minority of patients who will run out of money, here is the way the process would work:

- Employer-based: each company will develop its own plan that identifies financial responsibility regarding MSA overspend. For example, the employee may have a $1,000 maximum out-of-pocket allowance and the employer pays for the remaining expenses incurred within that year.

- Medicare: The federal government would have a program that subsidizes any overspending by Medicare patients.

Point to ponder: The average sixty-five-year-old working in my office will receive $10,340 per year in their MSA account. This is my actual cost for 2010 outpatient premium for one of my employees.

"What happens to the money in my account if I lose my job?"

—Stella Y., Yukon, OK

The money in your medical savings account will remain in your account and belongs solely to you. It does not belong to your employer; it is yours and will stay with you even if you change jobs.

"I predict there will be people who don't go to the doctor when they need to because they will be afraid of running out of money. What about them?"

—Kyle S., Des Moines, WA

There may well be patients who fear using up the funds in their MSA. Under the current system individuals have an even stronger incentive NOT to go to the doctor, buy medication, or have testing done because large co-pays or deductibles are cost-prohibitive. Under the new system, out-of-pocket spending goes away; simply swipe the MSA card and the amount will be deducted from your account. Financial barriers for medical care will cease. Patients will enjoy the unparalleled freedom of choosing their health-care plan without fear of co-pays and deductibles while still retaining the financial incentives to avoid overspending.

"Not everyone has the capacity to manage their own accounts. What about them?"

—Darcy D., Minneapolis, MN

First, let me just say that it is insulting to the majority of Americans to assume we are incapable of managing our own accounts. How many people in this country do not have checking accounts, savings accounts, monthly bills, driver's licenses, or the ability to decide if they can afford a steak or hamburger? If you need assistance or simply don't want to make the decisions, your physician should be able to manage your healthcare for you. If not, find another physician who has your best interests at heart. Guardians, spouses, friends, and family members will be another valuable management source. REMEMBER: ALL TREATMENTS AND TESTS WILL STILL REQUIRE A PHYSICIAN'S ORDER.

"How does the plan work with Medicare?"

—Jean W., Mantachie, MS

Medicare is already divided into Part A (Hospitalization) and Part B (Outpatient). The Part A premium is currently paid by the Social Security Administration and this part will not change. However, under our plan, the funds for Part B will go into your MSA account. Two positive changes: you will no longer need to buy supplemental health insurance AND the free market will drive down costs so your dollars will go further. The valid fear many senior citizens currently have, that doctors will not accept Medicare patients, will cease to exist. Medicare patients will have the same buying power as the privately insured. How about that great news?

"How will your program help the uninsured?"

—Karen G., New York City, NY

As a general rule, I restate the position that healthcare costs across the board will be more affordable. Thus, government-subsidized programs will be able to help more individuals at a lower overall cost. The MSA plan will allow the government to subsidize low-income families on a graduated basis.

"Without the insurance company keeping tabs on quality, how will I know if I have a good doctor?"

—Luis M., San Antonio, TX

The same way you know now. Being a "yes-man" to insurance companies does not make a physician a good doctor—far from it! You need a doctor to be an advocate for you, not to agree to treatments that are determined by big business. Insurance regulations are not a meaningful reflection of quality healthcare.

"What happens to the money in my account if I die?"

—Charles C., Philadelphia, PA

The state and federal politicians will have to duke it out to determine which party ultimately gets it, but the general idea is that if you pass away and have a remaining balance in your MSA, it will be returned to the government to fund the poor and underinsured.

"I have a chronic condition and will likely use up the money in my MSA faster than a healthier person. Isn't it unfair that I could potentially have to pay out-of-pocket while these people accumulate thousands of dollars in their account? "

—Brian P., San Jose, CA

How is your example different from the current system? Chronically ill folks spend a lot more money in the form of deductibles and co-pays already. Under the new system, because medical costs across the board will be less, out-of-pocket expenses will be reduced. It is not a stretch to state that "zero" out-of-pocket expenses are a reasonable expectation. Remember, under our new plan the money in the account can only be accessed for legitimate medical treatment so other than an added sense of security, a healthy person has no unfair advantage.

"Who can put money into the MSA account?"

—Christen S., New Prague, MN

ANYONE: Employers, individuals, family members, friends, government entities, etc. Wouldn't it be great if foundations and other organizations would contribute, too?

"Who decides where to put the money?"

—Sharon G., Kansas City, MO

You do. The only stipulation is that it be to a federally insured financial institution. The funds could be moved from one institution to another. Naturally, they would be placed in an interest-bearing account and conceivably would inspire financial institutions to compete against one another to offer higher interest rates.

"Does this program apply to illegal aliens?"

—Larry W., Hot Springs, AR

Individuals would have to have social security numbers to qualify for MSAs.

"What if I want to spend my money on cosmetic surgery or non-conventional medical care or therapies?"

—Mary B. , Denver, CO

There will always be a need for some type of regulation within the healthcare arena. The government would need to mirror, at least in part, the guidelines currently mandated for existing HSAs. Otherwise, vulnerable or misguided people would risk using up the money in their accounts on unnecessary medical care.

"Wouldn't a medical free market backfire?"

—Shaun G., Burnsville, MN

No. This is the United States, folks. A free market is based on checks and balances, not total deregulation. We expect quality and choice in nearly every facet of our lives. Why should we expect less from something as fundamental as our healthcare?

"Wouldn't this plan really cause just as much paperwork as you have now?"

—Anne M. , Oklahoma City, OK

Well…there will always be paperwork. My patients' health is my ultimate priority, and documenting and auditing their charts appropriately is the responsibility of any good doctor or medical professional. Having said that, under our plan there would be NO insurance billing, formularies, or quality reporting. This will reduce costs, in some cases drastically, for ALL employers, doctors, diagnostic centers, laboratories, medical suppliers, insurance companies, and numerous other goods and services. As a result of reducing their costs, yours will go down as well.

"Frankly, Dr. Brown, I am happy with the insurance company making lists of approved medical providers. Seeking out my medical provider would be just one more thing for me to do. Why should I care? After all, you are on my list."

—Jamie G., Oxford, MS

This may be one of the most common questions I've been asked. Flattery aside, the danger of the current system running doctors like me out of business is very real. You and I should both care that medical costs are inflated and tax our entire economic system with such an unnecessary burden. I am not an alarmist by nature, but after years of seeing first-hand the deterioration of healthcare, I am finally scared. Given a choice, I can't help but believe the majority of Americans would like to see more money in their paychecks and realize the benefits of more equitable costs and services.

"When the eagles are silent, the parrots begin to jabber."

—Winston Churchill

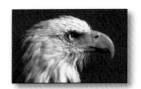

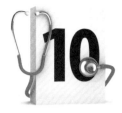

A Real Solution

Secrets do not have to be hidden away deep in the back of closets to find shelter from prying eyes. In fact, some of the best-kept secrets in healthcare are right in front of you, hidden in plain sight. It is my hope that as you turned the pages of this book any blinders you may have had melted away, leaving new understanding. Through expert conditioning, you may have been so accustomed to the current corrupt system that you didn't realize your rights have been taken away.

Charla, my patient, and I have spent the last year attempting to put on paper how the current system has failed us. Your money. My money. Waste to the tune of a trillion dollars a year.

Let me again state we should not retrofit the current system; we need a NEW system.

We cannot have a real solution unless we identify the problems. As you can see from reading these pages, the problems come from third parties, be it the government or insurance companies. They have too much control, and with control, there comes much power.

In an effort to control costs and increase profits, prices have been fixed, taking away the free market and along with it the long-held expectation Americans hold dear: freedom of choice. In most facets of our society, price fixing is illegal as it inhibits fair competition. Our statutes clearly state those companies, vendors, manufacturers, and other service providers cannot act in concert with one another to control or fix prices within a market. I am left thinking there are a lot of folks out there clearly not getting the memo!

As a result, overhead is rapidly increasing and sustainability is impossible to maintain. Let me repeat this statement: the current system is not sustainable. As the system gets more and more complex, there is more room for lobbyists, special interest groups, and private insurance providers to play games and manipulate. Have you ever gone a year without your personal insurance premiums rising?

It is time to take the control away from the government and insurance companies and give it to you, the customer or patient. After all, you are paying the bill. Remember the hardware store analogy? Competition works in every other avenue of American life, why not with healthcare?

Medical Savings Accounts Dr. Brown's Way addresses every single issue in health care today:

- Patients will continue to have the incentive not to spend money unnecessarily, making co-pays and deductibles obsolete.

- A free market will lower the actual costs of drugs, procedures, and doctor visits as patients will not want to run out of money.

- A free market will give medical providers the freedom to be creative in the services they provide, while also increasing the quality of care.

- The benefits of quality preventive treatments will be realized as patients no longer have the barrier of co-pays and deductibles, leading to less expensive hospitalizations and treatments down the road.

- Overhead of outpatient care will get close to nothing.

- Fraud will also go away as there are no longer false claims submitted to insurance companies.

- Physician overhead would decrease an average of 7 percent.

- Lower healthcare costs will make it easier to provide care for the poor and uninsured.

As a result, more money will be in your pocket and lead to a healthier economy.

Please join us in demanding your employer and legislators adopt this plan. It is not unreasonable to expect that

A Patient's Perspective

"Dr. Brown's plan can be achieved *without* a 2,409-page legislative bill. If the responsibility of spending money properly is in the hands of the customer or patient, most regulation would be unnecessary as patients and doctors can regulate themselves much better. This is not a new concept, but a time-proven facet of a democratic free market.

"We the People" of the United States of America have the capacity to demand healthcare reform. Further, it is not unreasonable to believe our healthcare costs should at least mirror those countries who offer similar quality.

We have a choice to make about healthcare today. We can choose to take back the right to make decisions that affect us; or, we can be complacent and let the powers that be continue to make fools of us.

Abraham Lincoln once said, "America will not be destroyed from the outside. If we falter and lose our freedoms, it will be because we have destroyed ourselves."

My name is Merlin Brown, and I am a medical doctor. Her name is Charla Sheffield, and she is my patient. Together, we have been equally frustrated, but the reality is, a year after we began this journey, we are now equally hopeful. Meaningful change can happen. It is up to us.

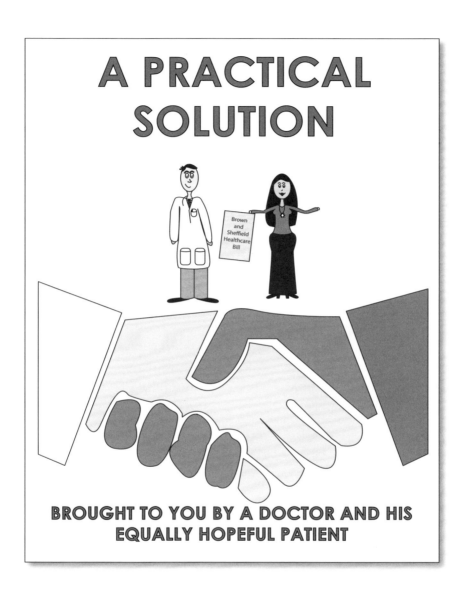

About the Authors

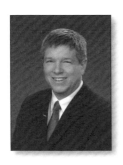 **Merlin Brown, MD**, was born in Tennessee but spent most of his growing-up years on a small farm in Wisconsin. After high school, he spent a year in France learning the language and working on his degree in French and then went on to prepare for Medical School. He graduated from Loma Linda University School of Medicine in 1990 and finished his residency in internal medicine in 1993. He currently is in private practice in a small internal medicine group in Edina, MN. Merlin is known for his compassionate medical care for adults of all ages and thrives on building long-term relationships with his patients. He has many outside interests, including building apartments and condominiums. He also has developed homes in Wisconsin for the mentally challenged. Merlin is an avid world traveler and in his leisure time he loves to garden and cook at his home in Minneapolis.

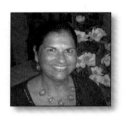 **Charla Sheffield** is a marketing execu-
tive and has been a patient of Dr. Brown's
since 1996. She is a cancer survivor and
has extensive patient experience at managing through the complexities of the
current healthcare system. She has an
executive certification in negotiation from the University
of Notre Dame, an MBA in marketing from the University
of Phoenix, and a BA in organizational management and
human relations from MidAmerica Nazarene University. Of
mixed heritage, she is a long-time youth mentor and advocate for Native American elders. She is active in her church,
an avid reader, and hospice volunteer. She lives in Minne-
sota with her husband, four children, two grandchildren,
two cats, and Bella the chiweenie. Formerly of General
Mills, Charla is currently a vice-president of marketing for a
top business-to-business media company.